THIS BOOK BELONGS TO

_____

I have put it off long enough. I am ready to calm the fuck down. Right here, right now.

If found, please . . .

return ◯

shred ◯

burn ◯

do yourself a favor
and buy your own
f**king copy ◯

Also by Sarah Knight

The Life-Changing Magic of Not Giving a F**k

Get Your Sh*t Together

Get Your Sh*t Together Journal

You Do You

Calm the F**k Down

F**k No!

Calm the F**k Down Journal

Practical ways to stop worrying
and take control of your life

SARAH KNIGHT

Quercus

Stop freaking out about
shit you can't control

and

Enable yourself to make
rational decisions

so you can

Solve problems instead
of making them worse.

What it is

This journal is based on a book I wrote about dealing with anxiety – from the white noise of what-ifs to the white-hot terror of a full-blown crisis. As such, you'd be forgiven for thinking I'm the world's biggest asshole for titling them as I have, since everyone knows that the first entry on a long list of Unhelpful Things to Say to a Person Experiencing Anxiety is "Calm the fuck down."

But they are also, respectively, a book and a journal about problems – we've all got 'em – and calming down is exactly what you need to do if you want to solve 'em. It is what it is. So if it keeps you from wanting to murder the messenger, know that throughout these pages I'm saying "Calm the fuck down" the same way I said "Get your shit together" in the *New York Times* bestselling book (and journal!) of the same name – not to shame or criticize you, but to offer motivation and encouragement.

I promise that's all I'm going for. (And that I'm not the world's biggest asshole; that honor belongs to whoever invented the vuvuzela.)

Who it's for

Before we dive into all of that anxiety-reducing, problem-solving goodness, I want you to know that I understand the difference between anxiety, the mental illness, and anxiety, the temporary state of mind. I understand it because I myself happen to possess a diagnosis of Generalized Anxiety and Panic Disorder. (Write what you know, folks!)

So although a profanity-riddled self-help book is no substitute for professional medical care, if you picked up the *Calm the Fuck Down Journal* because you're perennially, clinically anxious like me, in it you will find plenty of tips, tricks, and techniques to help you manage that shit, which will allow you to move on to the business of solving the problems that are feeding your anxiety in the first place.

But maybe you don't have – or don't realize you have, or aren't ready to admit you have – anxiety, the mental illness. Maybe you just get temporarily anxious when the situation demands it (see: the white-hot terror of a full-blown crisis). Never fear! This journal will provide you with ample calamity management tools for stressful times.

Plus maybe some tips, tricks, and techniques for dealing with that thing you don't realize or aren't ready to admit you have.

Just sayin'.

How to use it

The *Calm the Fuck Down Journal* is a place for you to ask and answer questions that may have been swirling around your brain like minnows on a meth bender, but that you haven't really confronted before – at least not in a logical, rational, effective way.

I devised a fun diagnostic quiz to start you off, and several exercises that are unique to the journal. Exciting! Plus you'll get quick-and-dirty introductions to various theories, methods, and strategies from the original book, and lots of space for you to take them to the next level.

Tools = my job. Using them = your job. Sound good?

The *Calm the Fuck Down Journal* will help you learn how to stop dwelling on unlikely outcomes in favor of creating more likely ones. How to plow forward rather than agonize backward. And crucially, how to separate your anxiety about what might occur from the act of handling it when it does occur.

Along the way, please remember: I'm not here to invalidate or minimize your anxiety or your problems. I just want to assist you in dealing with them, and calming the fuck down is the first step.

Let's get started.

SHIT THAT HASN'T HAPPENED YET

The What-ifs

A massive part of anyone's anxiety stems from Shit That Hasn't Happened Yet, or what I call "the what-ifs." So to kick things off, I'd like to ask you a few questions:

- How many times a day do you ask yourself *What if?* As in: *What if X happens? What if Y goes wrong? What if Z doesn't turn out like I want/need/expect it to?*

- How much time do you spend worrying about something that hasn't happened yet? Or about something that not only hasn't happened, but probably won't?

- And – moving on to Shit That Has *Already* Happened – how many hours have you wasted freaking out about something that has already happened (or avoiding it, as a quiet panic infests your soul) instead of just dealing with it?

In case you're wondering, my answers are: Too many, too much, and a LOT.

If yours are too, then this journal is *definitely* for you.

Keep reading!

When we're finished, the next time you come down with a case of the what-ifs – and whether they remain theoretical anxieties (Shit That Hasn't Happened Yet) or turn into real, live problems that need solvin' (Shit That Has Already Happened) – instead of worrying yourself into a panic attack, crying the day away, punching a wall, or avoiding things until they get even worse, you'll have learned to replace the open-ended nature of that unproductive question with one that's much more logical, realistic, and actionable.

OKAY,
NOW WHAT?

SHIT HAPPENS.

It's how you handle it that
makes all the difference.

In this part of the journal, I'll introduce the Four Faces of Freaking Out and we'll figure out which ones are most applicable to you and your life.

We'll also study the evolution of a freakout:

- How it happens
- What it looks like
- What it costs you

And I'll outline a few other key concepts that will resurface as we go along, including:

- Mental decluttering
- Emotional puppy-crating
- Freakout funds
- Naming your tarantulas
- The One Question to Rule Them All

(You might want to bookmark that last one. It's important.)

The Four Faces of Freaking Out

_____

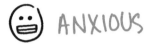 ANXIOUS

 SAD

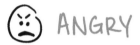 ANGRY

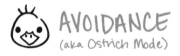 AVOIDANCE
(aka Ostrich Mode)

Some of us don't blink an eye when our septic tanks back up, but hyperventilate if Starbucks runs out of almond croissants. Others pull a Cool Hand Luke when the car gets towed or the test results come back positive, but reach our own personal DEFCON 1 when the cable goes out during *America's Next Top Model*. Freaking out manifests in different strokes for different folks. For some it's the openmouthed, panic-sweating countenance of a *Cathy* cartoon from the eighties ("Ack!"); but for others, freaking out is more about tears than tremors. Or black moods. Or blank stares.

And to top it all off – any one of us might experience a different form of freakout on a different day, for a different reason. Ain't life grand?

But generally speaking, most of us have a go-to freakout face. Mine is anxiety.

Time to figure out what yours is . . .

What's your freakout face?

_____

1. **You're stuck in traffic and late for an important meeting. What do you do?**
    a) Panic. I'm probably going to get fired, or at least scolded by my boss.
    b) I get depressed because I feel like I can't do anything right.
    c) Start cursing everyone on the road.
    d) Arrive late, don't go to the meeting at all, and try to avoid my boss for three days.
    e) Queue up another podcast and wait patiently.

2. **You're having a dinner party and the main course was a disaster. What's your first reaction?**
    a) My heart starts pounding. What is everyone going to eat?!?
    b) I'm so upset I might cry in front of my guests.
    c) Make a guttural noise and slam a bunch of pots and pans around.
    d) Pretend like everything is fine and hope everyone else does, too.
    e) Eh, it's not a big deal. We can order pizza.

3. You've been asked to give an important toast at a friend's wedding. How do you feel the morning of?
   a) Sick to my stomach with nerves.
   b) I can't believe they put their trust in me. I'm terrible at this stuff.
   c) I hate this kind of thing and I'm already in a bad mood.
   d) I . . . um . . . haven't exactly prepared.
   e) Fine. Why?

4. You think you messed up on a big exam. Results are in tomorrow. What's going through your head?
   a) Literally every question, over and over again, and I won't be sleeping tonight.
   b) I'm such a pathetic failure.
   c) I feel like screaming. I fucking blew it.
   d) Let's just say it's going to be a while before I even look at the results.
   e) I'll figure it out when the time comes.

5. The current state of world politics has you feeling mostly —
   a) Terrified for the future.
   b) Hopeless.
   c) Incandescent with rage.
   d) I can't think about it.
   e) I'm pretty Zen, tbh.

6. You're on vacation. The weather is ruining all your plans. How do you feel?
    a) Anxious about wasting money on this trip.
    b) This stuff always happens to me. I'm so tired of being disappointed all the time.
    c) I used my vacation days on this? Fuck, fuck, FUCK!
    d) I'm going to bed. For three days.
    e) Who wants to play Boggle?

7. You've had a weird rash for a while and you should go to the doctor.
    a) I'm going to die, aren't I?
    b) I'm gross. I don't even want to leave my house, let alone go to the doctor.
    c) Dammit, I don't have time for this shit.
    d) Yeah, I'll get on that sometime in the nonspecific future.
    e) It doesn't seem like a big deal, but okay, I'll make an appointment.

8. Work is stressful lately. What's your go-to coping mechanism?
    a) I don't have time to cope. I'm too busy freaking out about getting everything done.
    b) It's hard enough to get out of bed and go to work. There is no coping.
    c) I like to throw things at other things, such as "staplers" and "walls."
    d) I'm a big fan of "ignoring it and hoping it will go away."
    e) I just relax when I get home. Doesn't everybody?

9. Your sister brings her obnoxious boyfriend to your birthday party uninvited. How do you handle it?

   a) What if I say something and she makes a scene? This could go badly. It's giving me a headache just thinking about it.

   b) I'm just sad that she doesn't care about me enough to respect my birthday.

   c) Have a go at her and kick him out, consequences be damned.

   d) I'm not going to bring it up. Ever.

   e) That kind of shit doesn't really bother me.

10. If a tree falls in the forest, it —

   a) Makes you worried about getting hit by a falling tree.

   b) Makes you sad that a tree has died.

   c) Makes you angry about deforestation and climate change.

   d) Makes you unwilling to face the effects of deforestation and climate change.

   e) Makes no difference to your life whatsoever.

If you got mostly As . . . 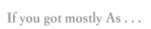 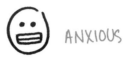 ANXIOUS

What it looks like: Anxiety comes in many forms, and for the uninitiated it can sometimes be hard to label. For example, you may think you've got a touch of food poisoning, when your upset stomach is actually due to anxiety. Or you might think you've been poisoned when really you're just having an old-fashioned panic attack. (Been there, thought that.)

Other indicators include but are not limited to: nervousness, headaches, hot flashes, shortness of breath, light-headedness, insomnia, indecision, the runs, and compulsively checking your email to see if your editor has responded to those pages you sent an hour ago. (And remember, you don't have to be diagnosed with capital-A Anxiety Disorder to experience lowercase-a anxiety. Plenty of calm, rational, almost-always-anxiety-free people go through occasional bouts of situational anxiety. Good times.)

Why it's bad: Apart from the symptoms I listed above, one of the most toxic and insidious side effects of being anxious is OVERTHINKING. It's like that buzzy black housefly that keeps dipping and swooping in and out of your line of vision, and every time you think you've drawn a bead on it, it changes direction. Up in the corner! No, wait! Over there by the stairs! Uh-oh, too slow! Now it's hovering three feet above your head, vibrating like the physical manifestation of your brain about to explode. WHERE DO YOU WANT TO BE, HOUSEFLY??? MAKE UP YOUR MIND.

Overthinking is the antithesis of productivity. I mean, have you ever seen a fly land anywhere for more than three seconds? How much could they possibly be getting accomplished in any given day?

What can you do about it? You need to Miyagi that shit. Focus. One problem at a time, one part of that problem at a time. And most important: one solution to that problem at a time.

I'll show you how.

If you got mostly Bs . . . 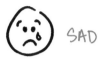 SAD

What it looks like: Weeping, moping, rumpled clothes, running mascara, the scent of despair, and heaving breathless, heaving breaths. It can also lead to a condition I call Social Media Self Pity, which is tiring not only for you, but also for your friends and followers. Cut it out, Ted. Nobody wants to watch you have an emotional breakdown in Garfield memes.

Why it's bad: Listen, I've got absolutely nothing against a good cry. You're worried that your childhood home is going to be bulldozed by evil city planners or that your hamster, Ping-Pong, might not make it out of surgery? By all means, bawl it out. I do it all the time. Catharsis!

Just try not to, you know, wallow. When worrying becomes wallowing – letting sadness overtake you for long periods of time – you've got bigger problems. Ongoing sadness is EXHAUSTING. You'll get less and less productive. And all of that can lead to feeling depressed and giving up on dealing with your shit altogether.

But to be clear, being sad – even for a messy, depressing stretch – is one thing. Having clinical depression is another. If you think you might not be merely sad, but fully in the grip of depression, I urge you to seek help beyond the pages of a book written by a woman whose literal job is to come up with new ways to work "fuck" into a sentence. And don't be ashamed about it.

What can you do about it? Patience, my pretties. We're gonna get you up and out of bed sooner rather than later. It's what Ping-Pong would have wanted.

If you got mostly Cs . . . 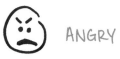 ANGRY

What it looks like: Apart from the yelling, screaming, and wishing poxes on people or setting fire to their prized possessions, those in the throes of anger experience unhealthy side effects such as rising blood pressure and body temperature, the desire to inflict physical violence and the injuries sustained upon doing so, splotchy faces, clenched jaws, and unsightly bulging neck tendons.

But an invisible – though no less damaging – result of an angry freakout is that it impedes good judgment. IT MAKES THINGS WORSE.

Why it's bad: In the age of smartphone cameras, every meltdown is a potential fifteen minutes of infamy. Do you want to wind up on the evening news spewing regrettable epithets or on Facebook Live destroying public property because you couldn't calm the fuck down? No, you do not.

What can you do about it? Well, you could take an anger-management class, but that doesn't sound very pleasant. I have a few stimulating alternatives I think you're going to like.

If you got mostly Ds . . . 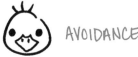 AVOIDANCE

aka Ostrich Mode

What it looks like: The tricky thing about Ostrich Mode is that you may not even realize you're doing it, because "doing it" is quite literally "doing nothing." You're just ignoring or dismissing warnings and pretending like shit isn't happening. Nothing to see here, folks! Head firmly in the sand.

Sometimes the 'strich stands alone – if you're merely putting off a mundane chore, that's pure, unadulterated avoidance. Other times, ostriching is the result of having already succumbed to anxiety, sadness, and/or anger. In those moments it feels like your brain is a pot of boiling lobsters, and if you can just keep the lid tamped down tightly enough, maybe you'll never have to confront their silent screams.

Why it's bad: Un-dealt-with shit begets more shit. Ignoring a jury summons can lead to fines, a bench warrant, and a misdemeanor on your permanent record. Pretending like you haven't developed late-life lactose intolerance can lead to embarrassing dinner party fallout. And refusing to tend to that pesky wound you got while chopping down your Christmas tree may mean spending the New Year learning to operate a prosthetic hand better than you operate an axe. And while I concede that wilfully ignoring whatever shit may be happening to you is a shrewd means of getting around having to deal with it – guess what?

If your worries have sent you into Ostrich Mode, you haven't actually escaped them. They'll be sitting right outside your hidey-hole the next time you lift your head. (Hi, guys. Touché.) Avoidance means NEVER, EVER SOLVING YOUR PROBLEM.

What can you do about it? Great question. Just by asking, you're already making progress.

If you got mostly Es . . .

Either you're deeply committed to lying to yourself, or you're actually in pretty good shape already, pal. Figure out which one it is and then either re-take the quiz or re-gift the journal to a friend. Sharing is caring!

And if you got a healthy mix of all the fucking letters . . .

Then you REALLY need this journal. And maybe a few spare pens. I have a feeling you're going to go through some ink.

So, how do you feel about your quiz results? Were they surprising? Or did you already know you were a specific kind of freaker-outer?

Use the next few pages to write down your thoughts, including symptoms of your personal freakouts, the effect they have on your life, and anything else you think is important at this stage. (Journaling is proven to help ease anxiety. Hey, don't take it from me – take it from SCIENCE!)

Good work on the journaling. (I hope it's starting to help; otherwise this is going to be no fun for either of us.)

Now that you know what your freakouts look like, let's look at how they happen:

EVOLUTION OF A FREAKOUT:

WHAT-IF
↓
WORRY
↓
INACTION
↓
FREAKOUT!

You start with a WHAT-IF – those pernicious little thoughts that fly into your head unbidden. They might be rooted in a real-life scenario, such as a party you're planning (*What if more people show up than RSVP'd? What if I didn't buy enough hot dogs?*); or they may be really far out, existential what-ifs (*What if I'm wasting my life in a career I don't love? What if I'm growing apart from my best friend?*).

Either way, you're beginning to get WORRIED.

Did you know that "worrying" has two separate but related meanings? In addition to the act of anxiously fretting about your problems, "worrying" also means constantly fiddling with something, rubbing at it, tearing it open, and making it worse.

It's like noticing that your sweater has a dangling thread, maybe the beginnings of a hole. And it's natural to want to pull on it. You're getting a feel for the problem, measuring its potential impact. (*How bad is it already? What can I do about it?*)

But if you keep pulling – and then tugging, yanking, and fiddling – and if you DON'T TAKE ACTION to fix it, suddenly you're down a whole sleeve, you're freaking out, and both your state of mind and your sweater are in tatters.

Congrats, now you're FREAKING OUT!

When you get into this state of mind, you're not just worrying about something; you're actually *worrying it*. And in both senses, it makes your problem worse. That's how it happens.

So how can you stop worrying? I'm so glad you asked. Behold!

THE NoWORRIES METHOD

Step 1:

CALM THE FUCK DOWN

Step 2:

AND DEAL WITH IT.

Mental decluttering

The NoWorries Method is based on the same concept that anchors all of my work: mental decluttering. Just like the physical decluttering made popular in recent years by Japanese tidying expert and author of *The Life-Changing Magic of Tidying*, Marie Kondo, mental decluttering has two steps:

DISCARDING and ORGANIZING

The difference is, my version of discarding and organizing happens entirely in your mind, not in your drawers or closets or garage. And the two steps of mental decluttering align not at all coincidentally with the two steps of the NoWorries Method.

Step 1: **DISCARD** your worries (aka calm the fuck down)

Step 2: **ORGANIZE** your response to what's left (aka deal with it)

That's it. Discard, then organize. And the way you begin is by looking at whatever problem you're worried about and asking yourself a very simple question.

CAN I CONTROL IT?

This, right here, is the key to the kingdom. Just like Marie Kondo asks you to decide if a material possession brings joy before you discard it, or like I ask you to decide if something annoys you before you stop giving a fuck about it, asking "Can I control it?" is the standard by which you'll measure whether something is worth your worries – and what, if anything, you can do about it.

The One Question to Rule Them All will stop those what-ifs from becoming worries, or at least stop the worries from becoming fully-fledged freakouts.

Now, take a second and flip back to page 12. Go ahead, I'll wait.

· · ·

That's right. It's not the what-if, the worry, or the actual bad shit that is going to make or break you. It's what you CAN or CANNOT do about it that really matters.

And then, HOW you proceed.

Oh, also, how your emotional puppies proceed.

Meet your emotional puppies

One of the things you can control right away in any given situation is your emotional response. So what does that have to do with puppies?

Well, I submit that emotions are *like* puppies. Sometimes they're purely fun and diverting; sometimes they're comforting or distracting; sometimes they just peed on your mother-in-law's carpet and aren't allowed in the house anymore. In any case, puppies are good for short periods of time until you have to get something accomplished, and then you need to coax them into a nice, comfy crate because you cannot – I repeat: CANNOT – deal with your shit while those little fuckers are on the loose. It's the same with emotions.

To be clear: It's okay to have emotions. It's even okay to freak out a little bit. But when your emotional puppies (emuppies?) are running amok, it's time to lock 'em up and, at least temporarily, misplace the key.

Now, crate your emotional puppies!

First, acknowledge the emotion – be it anxiety, anger, sadness, or one of their many tributaries (e.g., fear). Grant it a reasonable visitation period in which to healthily acknowledge its existence and let it wear itself out with a short burst of activity.

Then, mentally pick it up by the scruff of the neck and exile it while you get to work on solving the problems that brought it out to play in the first place.

If you practice mindfulness, you might know this trick as "Teflon mind," so termed because negative thoughts aren't allowed to stick. I think the puppy analogy is more inviting than the image of an eight-inch frying pan anywhere near your skull, but tomayto, tomahto.

And remember: in the same way that you can lock those rascals up, you can also let them back out whenever you want. Whenever you must. Whenever their precious puppy faces will make you feel better, not worse.

Woof.

Now, where were we before the puppies reared their heads?

Oh yes, remember that party you're hosting? You were worried about more people showing up than RSVP'd and running out of food.

Can you control it?

Yep! Just run out and grab an extra pack of dogs, and throw them in the freezer if they don't get eaten. By taking action – tying a knot in that loose thread – you can DISCARD this worry and prevent it from destroying your metaphorical sweater.

How about hating your job? Sure, maybe you can't change it right away, but there's nothing stopping you from Googling job postings, grad school courses, or a nice hypnotist who could help you out in a pinch.

The point is, it doesn't matter precisely what your what-ifs are – only that they exist and they're occupying some/a lot/too much of your mental space on any given day, unraveling your brain bit by bit.

To survive and thrive in these moments, you need to ACKNOWLEDGE what's happened, ACCEPT the parts you can't control, and ADDRESS the parts you can.

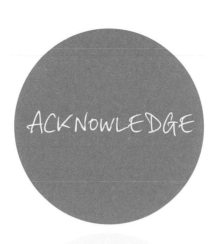

ACKNOWLEDGE

ACCEPT

ADDRESS

Think back over the last few weeks/months/years. What were three of your biggest freakouts? Make a list here:

1.
....

....

....

....

2.
....

....

....

....

3.
....

....

....

....

Could any of these have been averted by acknowledging the problem, accepting what you couldn't control, and addressing what you could? Use the next few pages to write about this stuff, with the One Question to Rule Them All (*Can I control it?*) as your guide.

(PS When you're done with this exercise, it'll be time to learn about what all that freaking out has COST YOU – and how you can get it back. Good times!)

Worrying is a waste
of your precious time,
energy, and money.

And worrying about
things you CAN'T
CONTROL is the
biggest waste of all.

Freakout funds

In *The Life-Changing Magic of Not Giving a Fuck* I introduced the concept of "fuck bucks," which are the resources – time, energy, and money – that you spend on everything you care about, from activities and appointments to friends, family, and more. Conversely, you can choose to not spend those resources on things you don't care about. Managing them is called "making a Fuck Budget," a concept that is on track to become my most enduring legacy. A *Lemonade* for anti-gurus, if you will.

Since you don't fix what ain't broke, I carried fuck bucks and the budgeting thereof through to the next book, *Get Your Shit Together* – the premise being that you also have to spend time, energy, and/or money on things you MUST do, even if you don't really WANT to do them – like, say, going to work so you can earn money so you can pay your rent. In the epilogue, I warned (presciently, as it turns out) that "shit happens" and "you might want to reserve a little time, energy, and money for that scenario, just in case."

Freakout funds are the fuck bucks you access when shit happens.

You could spend them indulging in your anxiety, sadness, anger, or avoidance – or, and this is preferable – you could spend them calming the fuck down and dealing with the shit that caused said freakout.

TIME

Time has been in finite supply since, well, since the beginning. They're not making any more of it. Which means that eventually you're going to run out of time to spend doing everything including freaking out about or dealing with whatever is about to happen/is happening/just happened to you. Why waste it on the former when spending it on the latter would vastly improve the quality of your entire remaining supply of minutes?

ENERGY

You will also eventually run out of energy, because although Jeff Bezos is trying really hard, he has not yet programmed Alexa to suck out your mortal soul while you're sleeping and recharge you on Wi-Fi. At some point, you have to eat, rest, and renew the old-fashioned way and if the shit does hit the fan, you'll wish you'd spent less energy freaking out about it and had more left in the tank to devote to dealing with it.

MONEY

This one's more complex, since some people have a lot and some people have none, and everyone's ability to replenish their coffers varies. But if you're broke, then stress-shopping while you freak out about passing the bar exam is obviously poor form. Whereas if you've got a bottomless bank account, you might argue that cleaning out the J.Crew clearance rack is at least contributing to the improvement of your overall mood. I'm not one to pooh-pooh anyone's version of self-care, but all that money you spent on khaki short-shorts and wicker belts is definitely not solving the underlying problem of your LSAT scores. Hiring a tutor would probably be a better use of funds.

GOODWILL

This is what I call "the Fourth Fund." Unlike time, energy, and money, the goodwill account is not held by you. It is funded by the sympathy and/or assistance of others, and is theirs to dole out or withhold as they see fit. Your job is to keep your account in good standing by not being a fucking freakshow all the time.

Beware "Constant Crisis Mode"

It's human nature to commiserate on occasion. We all do it. When you're feeling overcome by the sheer magnitude of your personal misfortune, it's understandable to seek comfort and support from others. And when your friends, family, and colleagues see you in distress, their first reaction will probably be to give you that comfort and support.

But if you freak out all the time, about everything, you're spending heavily against your account of goodwill – and you're in danger of overdrawing it faster than they drain the aquarium after a kid falls into the shark tank, resulting in the classic Boy Who Cried Shark conundrum:

When you need that help and sympathy for something worthy, there may be none left.

So, remember those three big freakouts I asked you to write about? How much time, energy, money, and goodwill did you spend either FUELING your freakout or DEALING WITH the problem?

In the next few pages, write it all down, and look at where you wasted funds versus where you spent them wisely.

For example, I spent way too much time Googling "ringworm" this month when I could have been working on this journal. I had already spent time, energy, and money going to the doctor and getting medicine for it; the Googling only wasted time and gave me anxiety, which in turn drew heavily on the goodwill fund maintained by my husband. Oops.

(Oh, and if you don't have three big freakouts to journal about just yet, no problem. Those blank pages will be waiting for you when you need them.)

FREAKOUT #1

Time wasted:

....

....

....

Time spent wisely:

....

....

....

Energy wasted:

....

....

....

Energy spent wisely:

....

....

....

Money wasted:

....

....

....

Money spent wisely:

....

....

....

Goodwill wasted:

....

....

....

Goodwill spent wisely:

....

....

....

FREAKOUT #2

Time wasted:

Time spent wisely:

Energy wasted:

Energy spent wisely:

Money wasted:

....

....

....

Money spent wisely:

....

....

....

Goodwill wasted:

....

....

....

Goodwill spent wisely:

....

....

....

FREAKOUT #3

Time wasted:

....

....

....

Time spent wisely:

....

....

....

Energy wasted:

....

....

....

Energy spent wisely:

....

....

....

Money wasted:

....

....

....

Money spent wisely:

....

....

....

Goodwill wasted:

....

....

....

Goodwill spent wisely:

....

....

....

WELCOME TO THE FLIPSIDE !

NEWTON'S THIRD LAW OF MOTION:

For every action,
there is an equal and
opposite reaction.

Freakout Faces: The Flipsides

Okay, enough with the freaking out. Let's talk about where to go from there – or where to go so you never get there in the first place.

You don't have to have taken high school physics (which I didn't, as may become obvious from my forthcoming interpretation of Newton's Third Law of Motion) to understand the idea that you can counteract a bad thing with a good thing. Laughing is the opposite of crying. Deep breaths are the opposite of lung-emptying screams. The pendulum swings both ways, et cetera, et cetera.

Ergo, one simple route to calming down pre-, mid-, or post-freakout is to – cue Gloria Estefan – turn the beat around.

Whichever freakout face you may be wearing (or merely be in danger of wearing), you need to learn how to flip the script.

Sing it, Gloria!

Anxious and overthinking?

FOCUS: Which of these worries takes priority? Which can you actually control? Zero in on those and set the others aside. (A bit of a recurring theme throughout the journal.)

Sad and exhausted?

REPAIR WITH SELF-CARE: Treat yourself the way you would treat a sad friend in need. Be kind. Naps, chocolate, baths, cocktails, a *South Park* marathon; whatever relieves your funk or puts a spring back in your step and a giggle in your wiggle.

Angry and making shit worse?

PEACE OUT WITH PERSPECTIVE: When you're getting hot under the collar, visualize the consequences and adjust your attitude accordingly. Sometimes that means adjusting your physical state, too.

Avoiding and prolonging the agony?

ACT UP: Take one step, no matter how small, toward acknowledging your problem. Say it out loud. Write it in steam on the bathroom mirror. Fashion its likeness into a voodoo doll. If you can do that, you're on your way to calming the fuck down.

In *Calm the Fuck Down*, I give lots of examples of how I flip my own script. For example, if I'm feeling anxious about all of the things on my to-do list, I take ten minutes to focus on a mindless task (mine is pruning a giant bush in my yard with a pair of kitchen scissors) to give my brain a chance to rest.

What are some ways you could focus your energy to stave off or dial down your anxiety?

Revisit this list when you're feeling anxious. I guarantee it will help!

If you're sad, what are some ways you could repair with self-care? (Remember: think about what you might do for someone else in need.)

....

....

....

....

....

....

....

....

....

....

....

Hey, guess what? You don't have to wait until you're feeling down to give yourself a pick-me-up. Try practicing some form of self-care at least once a week and see if it improves your overall mood.

If you're feeling angry, one surefire way to burn off that excess energy is to engage in physical activity, which boosts serotonin (aka "the happiness hormone") and gives you time to cool down and get back to a peaceful state. I personally hate running, but naked cartwheels are fun.

Name some ways you could see yourself peacing out with physical activity.

How creative did you get? If the answer is "Not very," then I suggest you attempt a naked cartwheel as soon as possible and tell me it doesn't render you positively jolly.

Finally, if you're going full Ostrich Mode and avoiding your shit, you need to take some action. I like to bargain with myself: as in, I'm not allowed to avoid two things at once, so if I want to continue ostriching on one, I have to do the other.

What are some things you've been avoiding that are causing you stress? Write them out and make a deal with yourself to take action on half of them.

I see you, my little ostrich. And I see you trying. Good job!

What seems to be the problem?

You've recalled past freakouts and all the funds you spent (and wasted) on them. You've learned about the Flipsides of the Four Faces and listed some ways for you to get there.

So what comes next?

Why, all of your *new* anxiety, of course!

If you're in touch with your what-ifs, you probably have a good handle on the underlying problems behind your potential future freakouts. I hope you won't freak out about most of them, of course. But at least you know what's on tap.

Then again – what if you don't?

A lot of people wake up feeling *blah* and *blech* for no reason. They can't pinpoint the source of their anxiety, sadness, or whatnot – and that is because they have not read this journal and do not know how to name their tarantulas.

Yes, you read that correctly.

Naming your tarantulas

There is a reason for your anxiety. A what-if behind your worry. And the sooner you name it, the sooner you're in a better position to calm the fuck down and deal with it.

To wit: I often think of my anxiety like a herd of giant spiders lurking in the shadows. (If you want to know the full story behind that, I'm afraid you'll have to read the original *Calm the Fuck Down* in its entirety.) I know it's there, but I can't see it and I certainly can't DO anything about it if I can't pin it down, can I? If I continue down this mental path, eventually I get so overwhelmed that I just start mumbling "Everything is a tarantula" under my breath until I short circuit.

But the fact is, everything is NOT a hidden tarantula. Everything is right out there in the open, with a name and a form of its own. Why did you wake up in an unspecified panic this morning? Maybe you have a deadline approaching. Or your parents are coming to visit. Why can't you fall asleep at night? Perhaps you're planning a big event, or you can't remember if you paid the phone bill.

Consider naming your tarantulas as the first step toward forcing them out in the open and dealing with them.

In other words: ACKNOWLEDGE the problem so you can ACCEPT and ADDRESS it.

Let's give it a shot.

My Tarantulas

I'm giving you a few more blank pages so you can come back and name future tarantulas as they pop up. (Figuratively, of course.)

Pick a category, any category!

Once you have a handle on your what-ifs and worries, and you've named the anxiety that's keeping you up at night, you can start to work on managing all of it. For that, I have a system.

THE SARAH KNIGHT SHITSTORM SCALE

Category 1: HIGHLY UNLIKELY

Category 2: POSSIBLE BUT NOT LIKELY

Category 3: LIKELY

Category 4: HIGHLY LIKELY

Category 5: INEVITABLE

If you've read any of my other books, you know I love to prioritize based on urgency. Anxiety is no different. If you're going to worry about shit (and we both know you are), at least you could be worrying about shit that's actually going to happen instead of stuff that exists only in your head or, like, several years down the line.

To that end, I give you: the PROBOMETER.

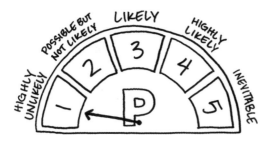

It's like an anemometer that measures the wind speed for hurricanes (also conveniently categorized by levels 1–5), but instead it measures the PROBABILITY of your PROBLEMS coming to pass.

Get it?

It doesn't matter what kind of what-if it is – big, small, serious, silly, frequent, or rare. The probometer doesn't care; all it asks is "How likely is this problem to occur?"

And all you have to do is answer. Then you can begin sorting your worries into neat mental piles. DISCARD the ones about shit that's unlikely to happen and ORGANIZE your response to what's left.

(Mental decluttering – I'm telling you, it's the tits.)

Pop quiz!

Forget about freakouts past. Name up to five what-ifs swirling inside your head RIGHT NOW:

1. ....

2. ....

3. ....

4. ....

5. ....

Next, use your probometer to categorize them. If they land at a 1 or a 2 on the Shitstorm Scale, do you see why you can worry about them less? Will you?

WHAT-IF #1

Category:

....

Can I worry about it less? Will I?

....

....

....

....

....

....

....

....

....

....

*Doesn't it feel good to think about your problems logically
and rationally? When in doubt, consult your probometer!*

Category:

Can I worry about it less? Will I?

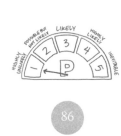

WHAT-IF #3

Category:

Can I worry about it less? Will I?

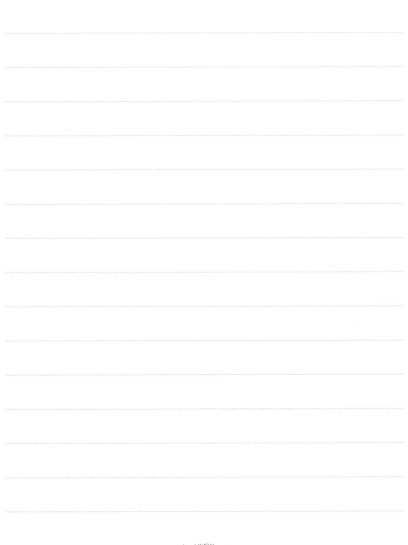

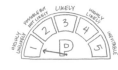

Category:

Can I worry about it less? Will I?

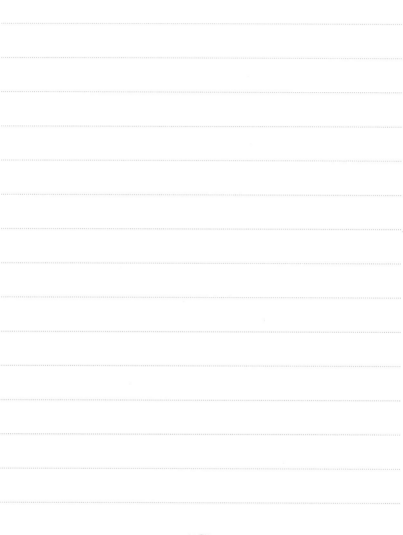

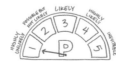

Category:

Can I worry about it less? Will I?

What's your status?

Once you have logically, rationally determined whether a what-if is a probable shitstorm, a useful follow-up question is **"How soon is it going to land?"**

There are three levels of urgency.

OUTLYING

IMMINENT

TOTAL

OUTLYING

An outlying shitstorm not only hasn't happened, you can't even be sure if it will. Theoretically, these should be the easiest to stop worrying about because they are both unlikely and distant – low pressure and low priority. Ironic, since low-pressure situations are what create legit rainstorms, but what can I say? Metaphors and the anti-gurus who employ them are imperfect.

Examples of outlying shitstorms:

- You might lose the election next year.
- You might not get promoted as fast as you wanted to.
- You might hurt yourself training for a marathon.
- You might never hear back from that girl you met at the bar.
- You might not lose the weight in time for the class reunion.
- You might follow in your parents' footsteps and need cataract surgery someday.
- You might get beaten to that patent by a fellow inventor.

IMMINENT

Imminent shitstorms also haven't happened yet, but they're more solidly formed and you're likely to know if and when they'll hit. You still might be able to prevent an imminent shitstorm, but if not, at least you can prep for impact and mitigate the fallout.

Examples of imminent shitstorms:

- You might lose the election *tomorrow*.
- You might not hit your 5p.m. deadline.
- You might fail your history exam on Monday.
- You might get in trouble for that inappropriate joke you just made in the meeting.
- You might not qualify for the mortgage.
- You might miss your tight connection in Philly.
- If she sees you leaving on the way in, your sister might find out you slept with her boyfriend.

TOTAL

A total shitstorm is one that is already upon you. You might've seen it coming when it was still imminent, or it may have appeared out of nowhere like some twelve-year-old YouTuber who has more followers than Islam and Christianity combined. It matters not whether the effects of the storm would be considered mild or severe (by you or anyone else) – it's here, and you have to deal with it. Whether the shitstorm is a Highly Unlikely Category 1 or an Inevitable 5 – if it hasn't happened yet, you can worry about it less urgently than if it's just about to or if it just did.

Examples of total shitstorms:

- You got red wine on your wedding dress.
- You got red wine on someone else's wedding dress.
- You received a scary diagnosis.
- Your company downsized you.
- Your car got towed.
- You lost a bet. A big bet.
- Your kid broke his leg.
- Your wife told you she's pregnant…with someone else's baby.

Pop quiz, part two!

Go back to those what-ifs from page 82:

1.

2.

3.

4.

5.

You already admitted to yourself how likely (or unlikely) they are to happen. If they are likely, then how soon do you really need to start worrying about them? Are they **OUTLYING, IMMINENT,** or **TOTAL**? Figure it out in the space provided.

WHAT-IF #1

Category:

Status:

WHAT-IF #2

Category:

....

Status:

....

....

WHAT-IF #3

Category:

....

Status:

....

....

WHAT-IF #4

Category:

....

Status:

....

....

Category:

Status:

OKAY, NOW WHAT?

I hope you're starting to see the big picture here, which is that your anxiety and the factors that cause it are manageable. (Or at least more manageable than they have been so far – I'm neither a doctor nor a miracle worker.)

Frankly, a bunch of this shit is unlikely to happen at all. You can prevent some of it and mitigate the effects of some of the rest. And some of it (those pesky Category 5s) is coming down the pike whether you like it or not.

What you can do to help yourself is use logical techniques to break down your worries and sort them into much smaller piles – those that are urgent, less urgent, or unworthy of your freakout funds at all.

You can DISCARD some and ORGANIZE your response to what's left.

How do you do that?

Come on . . . you know this . . .

CAN I CONTROL IT?

Exactly! And there are different kinds of control you may or may not be able to exert on any given situation. It's a sliding scale, and you'd be well served to understand the nuances.

Out of your hands

These are the things you can't control at all – such as the weather, other people's actions, the number of hours in a day, and the number of chances your boyfriend is going to give you before he gets sick of your *What if he's cheating on me* bullshit and dumps you anyway because you're needy and untrusting.

Make a contribution

You can't control the larger underlying problem, but you can do your part to minimize its effects. For example, in terms of the weather, you can't control the rain, but you can control *whether* or not you suffer its effects to the fullest if you bring an umbrella. You can't control the number of hours in a day, but you can control *whether* you spend too many of them watching online contouring tutorials instead of hand-washing your delicates like you should be. And you can't control Randy's ultimate level of tolerance for your "WHO IS SHE???" comments on his Facebook page, but you can control *whether* you keep using your fingers to tap out those three little words. (Or you could just break up with Randy because, let's face it, where there's smoke there's fire.)

Under your influence

This stuff, you can *heavily influence* if not completely control – such as "not oversleeping," by way of setting an alarm. Is it possible that something will prevent your alarm from going OFF (like a power outage or a mouse gnawing through the wire), or you from heeding its siren song (like accidentally pressing off instead of SNOOZE)? Sure, but that's a Category 1 Highly Unlikely Shitstorm and you know it. Or . . . am I to infer from this line of questioning that you don't really *want* to calm the fuck down?

Uh-huh. Carry on.

Complete control

This is shit you are always 100 percent in control of, such as "the words that come out of your mouth" and "whether or not you are wearing pants."

Before we tackle your own what-ifs, let's road test The One Question to Rule Them All on other people's problems. The following examples from the original *Calm the Fuck Down* book were adapted from an anonymous survey wherein I asked people what shit they were worried about these days. In the book, I answered them, but here, that's your job. (And if you own the book, no peeking! You shouldn't have to anyway, if you've been paying attention.)

If this were your problem, could you control it?*

What if I tell my bestie, Rachel, what I really think of her new bangs and she never forgives me?

Can I control it? (If so, what kind of control?)

What if I accidentally shout another woman's name in bed with my new girlfriend?

Can I control it? (If so, what kind of control?)

What if rumors of a union dispute come to pass and force the cancellation of that monster truck rally next Wednesday that I was all excited about?

Can I control it? (If so, what kind of control?)

What if something bad happens to people I give incorrect directions to?

Can I control it? (If so, what kind of control?)

What if I laugh so hard I pee my pants during my friend's stand-up gig?

Can I control it? (If so, what kind of control?)

....

....

....

....

I'm happy and in a good relationship, but what if we wait too long to get married and never have kids?

Can I control it? (If so, what kind of control?)

....

....

....

....

What if I'm failing as an adult?

Can I control it? (If so, what kind of control?)

....

....

....

....

What if I choose not to go home and visit my family this weekend and something bad happens to them and then I regret it forever?

Can I control it? (If so, what kind of control?)

....

....

....

....

* My answers can be found on pp. 190–91

Now let's do you! Go back one more time to those what-ifs from page 82:

1. ....

2. ....

3. ....

4. ....

5. ....

If any of these is a category 1 or 2, you shouldn't be worrying about them anyway – but just for the sake of argument, I want you to look at all of them and ask yourself *Can I control it?*

If the answer is yes, what steps can you take to prevent or mitigate the shitstorm in question?

(If the answer is no – hold that thought. We'll get to those in just a bit.)

Category:

Status:

Can I control it? (if so, how?):

Category:

Status:

Can I control it? (if so, how?):

Category:

Status:

Can I control it? (if so, how?):

Category:

Status:

Can I control it? (if so, how?):

Category:

Status:

Can I control it? (if so, how?):

If the answer is no,
this is how you let it go

Can you control it (or aspects of it) – yes or no? You already have the answers.

Okay, but how do I get from understanding that worry is pointless to actually not worrying?

Excellent question.

Once you **ACKNOWLEDGE** the problem, you begin to let go of your worries about said problem by **ACCEPTING** the things you can't control.

ACKNOWLEDGE

ACCEPT

ADDRESS

Reality check, please!

Please note: I am not using the word "acceptance" in the sense that you're supposed to suddenly become happy about whatever shit is about to happen or has happened that you can't control. It's totally understandable – especially in the short term – to be very fucking upset by shit we can't control, as Ross was when Rachel broke up with him on *Friends* using the very words "Accept that."

But if you've been dumped, duped, or dicked over, facts are facts. Continuing to spend time, energy, and/or money being anxious, sad, or angry about it (or avoiding it) is a waste of freakout funds. Girl, don't act like you don't know this. We've been over it multiple times.

So for the purposes of this journal, I'm using the word "accept" to mean "understand the reality of the situation."

That's not so hard, is it? If you can accept that the sky is blue and water is wet and macarons are disappointing and borderline fraudulent as a dessert, you can accept the things you can't control.

HUZZAH!

Sarah Knight, dropping commonsense knowledge bombs since 2015.

When you answer the One
Question to Rule Them All
with a *No*, you have already
accepted reality. You have
admitted that you can't control
something – it's that simple.

The path from what-ifs and worrying to calming the fuck down is a straight line from "things that exist in your imagination" to "things that exist in reality" and then "accepting those things as reality."

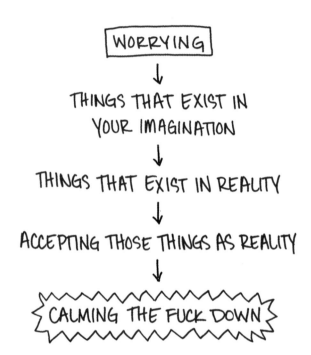

All that remains to complete
Step 1 of the NoWorries Method is to
DISCARD that unrealistic, unproductive
worry like the good little mental
declutterer I know you can be.

To do that, you have a couple of options.

Option 1: Just fucking let it go

You still think it's easier said than done? Fine. But I encourage you to consider everything we've talked about so far and apply your new tools and perspective on a case-by-case basis.

For example, if you're working those shitstorm categories like I taught you, you should be able to reduce your worry load immediately, and significantly.

If something is highly unlikely to happen, why are you worrying about it?

And if it's far off in the distance, why are you worrying about it NOW?

Oh, and is this something you can control? No? Hm. Then there's no reason you should be spending your precious time, energy, and money on it at all.

I'm not at all surprised that you couldn't just fucking let go of any of your worries before you picked up this journal – but I'd be really surprised if by now, you can't just fucking let go of, like, a bunch of them.

Option 2: Houdini that shit

True, you cannot count on becoming happy about the thing that, right now, has you very fucking upset.

But you CAN become happy (or calm or proactive, etc.), right now, about something else entirely – which in turn causes you to stop worrying about the original thing.

Ta-daaa! I call this technique "sleight of mind."

Just like sleight of hand enables a magician to perform his thrilling act, sleight of mind is how we'll make your worries disappear – at least temporarily, and maybe even for good.

(And don't come at me with "That's cheating!" I promised you tricks at the very beginning. You should really start taking me at my word.)

ANXIOUS? → FOCUS

SAD? → REPAIR WITH SELF-CARE

ANGRY? → PEACE OUT WITH PERSPECTIVE

AVOIDING? → ACT UP

Back on pages 66-71 I gave you a few tips on making your way to the Flipside. Here are four more, simple, elegant tricks you can tuck up your voluminous sleeve for when the worrying gets tough and the tough need to STOP WORRYING.

Focus

—————

Get down with O.P.P.

Other people's problems, that is. Maybe you don't have an on-call therapist – but you've got friends, family, neighbors, and the guy down at the post office with the beard that looks like it rehomes geese who got lost on their way south for the winter. Chat 'em up. Ask your sister how she's doing and listen to her shit. Release some of your anxiety by giving her advice that you should probably be taking your own damn self.

It's harder to stay anxious about any particular thing when you don't allow yourself the mental space to dwell on it – and a darn good way to accomplish that is by filling said space with conversation, human interaction, and other people's problems. How do you think I stay so calm these days? I spend all year giving you advice.

Make a list on the opposite page of people you could call or visit to help tame your anxiety – and why they could use your advice.

Other ways to reduce anxiety that I didn't invent but that have been known to work

- Deep breaths. In through the nose, out through the mouth.
- Yoga
- Sex
- Bubble baths
- Counting slowly to one hundred
- Magnesium supplements
- Adult coloring books

Repair with self-care

Laughter is the best medicine

Much like "Calm the fuck down," the phrase "Turn that frown upside down" is advice not often well received by a person who is midfreakout. I know that, but I'll say it anyway, because that shit works. For example, when I'm feeling utterly dejected, a certain someone's patented C + C Music Factory tribute dance/lip sync always brings me back from the brink.

If something has you down, seek help from things that reliably cheer you up. Cat pics. Videos of people coming out of anesthesia. Perhaps an aptly termed "feel-good movie"? Anything in the *Pitch Perfect* oeuvre applies. Even if this trick stops you worrying for only the length of one song (in my case, "Things That Make You Go Hmmm . . .") – you've stopped, haven't you? Progress!

Make a list on the opposite page of things that make you laugh. Don't be stingy!

Peace out with perspective

Plot your revenge

Hopefully they won't revoke my guru card for this one, but let's just say you live downstairs from Carl and his all-night drug parties, and every morning your anger rises just as he and his crew finally drop off into a cracked-out slumber. Instead of seething into your dark roast, you might consider perking up by mentally cataloguing the ways in which you could repay your neighbor's kindness.

No need to follow through – merely thinking about the mayhem you could visit upon your enemies is a terrific mood booster. Plus it helps you visualize an outlet for your anger and "slow your roll," so to speak. Twenty minutes spent plotting is twenty minutes you're not doing something else in a fit of rage that you may regret – and get in big trouble for – later.

Use the opposite page to dash off some ideas for THEORETICAL retaliation against whatever person, thing, organization, or concept gets your blood boiling. The more creative, the better!

Forms of revenge that are fun to think about

- Writing your enemy's phone number and a related "service" on the wall of a sketchy bar bathroom. Or, like, fifty sketchy bar bathrooms.

- Ordering a 4a.m. wakeup call to your enemy's hotel room

- Mailing your enemy a box of loose black pepper

- Filling your enemy's pants pockets with gum right before they go into the wash

Act up

Get alarmed

If you're putting something off – say, having "the talk" with your teenage son – use the alarm feature on your smartphone or watch to remind you about it ten times a day until you'd rather unroll a condom onto a banana than listen to that infernal jingle-jangle ONE MORE TIME. Even if you chicken out yet again, you'll have forced yourself to acknowledge the situation with every beep of your alarm, and that's half the battle.

(Actually, if you've been paying attention, it's one third of the battle. The middle third is accepting that you can't control a fifteen-year-old's libido, and the final third is addressing the part you can control – teaching safe sex – with prophylactics and phallic produce.)

Remember the stuff you made a deal with yourself to stop avoiding back on page 71? Write them out fresh below, set a week's worth of alarms for the first one on your list, do the damn thing, and repeat until complete.

Secret option C

"Just fucking let it go" and "sleight of mind" are two excellent paths forward to a calmer, happier you. Highly recommended. But depending on the person and worry and related shitstorm in question, these two methods alone are not always enough.

As such, it's time for me to make a confession. Despite its powerful cross-branding with my NotSorry Method from *The Life-Changing Magic of Not Giving a Fuck* and a very strong hashtag, the "NoWorries" Method may be a slight misnomer.

No worries – like actually zero? Ever? That's probably not strictly possible. Sometimes your probometer is in the shop and your worries remain omnipresent and all-consuming.

Sometimes you really just can't stop worrying or focus on other things.

It's okay, we can work with that.

Ladies and Gentlemen of the Worry, I give you . . .

Productive Helpful Effective Worrying
(P. H. E. W.)

Up to this point, our goal has been to discard worries about shit you can't control, saving your time, energy, and money for dealing with the shit you can. We've been **CONSERVING** freakout funds.

That's one way to do it.

If you can't bring yourself to discard your worries altogether, another way to calm the fuck down is to **CONVERT** those worries into productive, beneficial action – ensuring that any FFs you dole out in advance of a shitstorm are spent wisely.

They will (at least) help prepare you for surviving it; and (at best) help prevent it altogether.

That's what makes it *productive*, *helpful*, and *effective* worrying. The awesome acronym is just a side benefit.

Getting to PHEW

- Once a shitstorm has been classified and prioritized, the NoWorries Method dictates that you ask yourself, Can I *control* it?

- If the answer is no, ideally you ACCEPT that you can't control it, and discard said worry. That's Step 1: Calm the fuck down.

- If the answer is yes, I can control it, then YAY! You may proceed directly to Step 2: Deal with it, organizing your response.

- However, if the answer is "No, I can't control it, BUT I ALSO CAN'T STOP WORRYING ABOUT IT OR DISTRACT MYSELF WITH OTHER THINGS!" then it's time to do some Productive Helpful Effective Worrying.

If it's something you can't control but you're going to worry about it anyway, you might as well spend those freakout funds taking action to prepare for it. For example:

- **What if I fuck up my kids and turn them into bad people?**

  Action you could take: Spend your time, energy, and money being the best parent you, personally, can be. Read to your kids. Tell them you love them. Teach them to say please and thank you and not kick sand on me at the beach.

  Outcome: At some point how they turn out is on them, but you'll know you did your best.

- **What if I go bald?**

  Action you could take: Instead of wasting money on products that don't really work, invest in some really cool hats.

  Outcome: Either you keep your hair or you become Really Cool Hat Guy. Maybe both.

You can't stop worrying? Fine. Worry away! But make it count for something.

If you're thinking that PHEW sounds suspiciously like addressing something, you're not entirely wrong, but I consider it more of an in-between step on the ACKNOWLEDGE → ACCEPT → ADDRESS continuum. If you haven't accepted the reality of a potential shitstorm such that you can't just stop worrying about it, you're kind of stuck in a gray area. Plus, "addressing it" is really for Shit That Has Already Happened. Don't worry, we're getting there.

The PHEW files

What are some things you've wasted freakout funds worrying about when you could have used PHEW instead? How about some upcoming shitstorms that might be good candidates for PHEW-ing? Use the next few pages to get a handle on what PHEW means to YOU.

Go forth and discard!

We've done a post-mortem on some of your past freakouts. We've addressed some current what-ifs. You've got the tools, so it's time to put them to good use now and in the future. The next section of the journal is for you to come back to in your time of need.

- When you have a what-if you can't shake, write it down.

- Use your probometer.

- Prioritize by urgency.

- Ask yourself the One Question to Rule Them All.

- And if you can: DISCARD that worry.

It's not like there won't be more where that came from, so practice making room for the ones you *can* control.

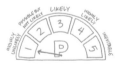

And if you get stuck, feel free to consult my handy "How do I calm the fuck down?" flowchart for assistance.

HOW DO I CALM THE FUCK DOWN?

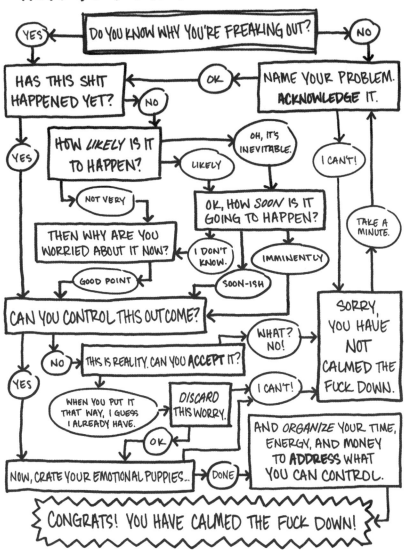

What-if:

....

....

Category:

....

....

Status:

....

....

Can I control it? (Or part of it)

....

....

If not, can I accept that reality, stop worrying about it,
and **CONSERVE** freakout funds?

....

....

If I can't stop worrying about it, can I **CONVERT** freakout funds to productive, helpful, effective worrying that will mitigate it?

....

....

....

....

All those things considered, can I stop worrying about it after all and move on to something else? If yes, great! If no, what's the plan?

....

....

....

....

....

....

....

What-if:

....

....

Category:

....

....

Status:

....

....

Can I control it? (Or part of it)

....

....

If not, can I accept that reality, stop worrying about it,
and **CONSERVE** freakout funds?

....

....

If I can't stop worrying about it, can I **CONVERT** freakout funds to productive, helpful, effective worrying that will mitigate it?

....

....

....

....

All those things considered, can I stop worrying about it after all and move on to something else? If yes, great! If no, what's the plan?

....

....

....

....

....

....

....

....

What-if:

....

....

Category:

....

....

Status:

....

....

Can I control it? (Or part of it)

....

....

If not, can I accept that reality, stop worrying about it,
and **CONSERVE** freakout funds?

....

....

If I can't stop worrying about it, can I **CONVERT** freakout funds to productive, helpful, effective worrying that will mitigate it?

All those things considered, can I stop worrying about it after all and move on to something else? If yes, great! If no, what's the plan?

What-if:

....

....

Category:

....

....

Status:

....

....

Can I control it? (Or part of it)

....

....

If not, can I accept that reality, stop worrying about it,
and **CONSERVE** freakout funds?

....

....

If I can't stop worrying about it, can I **CONVERT** freakout funds to productive, helpful, effective worrying that will mitigate it?

....

....

....

....

All those things considered, can I stop worrying about it after all and move on to something else? If yes, great! If no, what's the plan?

....

....

....

....

....

....

....

....

What-if:

....

....

Category:

....

....

Status:

....

....

Can I control it? (Or part of it)

....

....

If not, can I accept that reality, stop worrying about it,
and CONSERVE freakout funds?

....

....

If I can't stop worrying about it, can I **CONVERT** freakout funds to productive, helpful, effective worrying that will mitigate it?

....

....

....

....

All those things considered, can I stop worrying about it after all and move on to something else? If yes, great! If no, what's the plan?

....

....

....

....

....

....

....

....

What-if:

....

....

Category:

....

....

Status:

....

....

Can I control it? (Or part of it)

....

....

If not, can I accept that reality, stop worrying about it,
and **CONSERVE** freakout funds?

....

....

If I can't stop worrying about it, can I **CONVERT** freakout funds to productive, helpful, effective worrying that will mitigate it?

....

....

....

....

All those things considered, can I stop worrying about it after all and move on to something else? If yes, great! If no, what's the plan?

....

....

....

....

....

....

....

....

What-if:

Category:

Status:

Can I control it? (Or part of it)

If not, can I accept that reality, stop worrying about it,
and CONSERVE freakout funds?

If I can't stop worrying about it, can I CONVERT freakout funds to productive, helpful, effective worrying that will mitigate it?

....

....

....

....

All those things considered, can I stop worrying about it after all and move on to something else? If yes, great! If no, what's the plan?

....

....

....

....

....

....

....

....

What-if:

....

....

Category:

....

....

Status:

....

....

Can I control it? (Or part of it)

....

....

If not, can I accept that reality, stop worrying about it,
and **CONSERVE** freakout funds?

....

....

If I can't stop worrying about it, can I CONVERT freakout funds to productive, helpful, effective worrying that will mitigate it?

All those things considered, can I stop worrying about it after all and move on to something else? If yes, great! If no, what's the plan?

What-if:

....

....

Category:

....

....

Status:

....

....

Can I control it? (Or part of it)

....

....

If not, can I accept that reality, stop worrying about it,
and CONSERVE freakout funds?

....

....

If I can't stop worrying about it, can I **CONVERT** freakout funds to productive, helpful, effective worrying that will mitigate it?

....

....

....

....

All those things considered, can I stop worrying about it after all and move on to something else? If yes, great! If no, what's the plan?

....

....

....

....

....

....

....

What-if:

....

....

Category:

....

....

Status:

....

....

Can I control it? (Or part of it)

....

....

If not, can I accept that reality, stop worrying about it, and CONSERVE freakout funds?

....

....

If I can't stop worrying about it, can I **CONVERT** freakout funds to productive, helpful, effective worrying that will mitigate it?

....

....

....

....

All those things considered, can I stop worrying about it after all and move on to something else? If yes, great! If no, what's the plan?

....

....

....

....

....

....

....

SHIT
THAT HAS
ALREADY
HAPPENED

Much like its companion book, the *Calm the Fuck Down Journal* is approximately three quarters anxiety-assuaging and one quarter problem-solving. Because no matter how calm you get about it, there's usually still a mess that needs cleaning up.

You've already done a shit-ton of mental decluttering, Step 1: DISCARDING. You've rid yourself of so many unproductive worries that you should have a healthy supply of freakout funds left to move on to Step 2: ORGANIZING – aka dealing with whatever's left when the shit has well and truly hit the fan.

Let's get to it.

ACKNOWLEDGE

ACCEPT

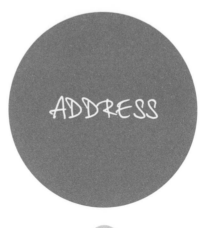

ADDRESS

The Three Principles of Dealing With It

Principle # 1: TAKE STOCK

Imagine you just landed in enemy territory and you have precious little time to assess the situation before it goes from bad to worse. You're going to have to grit your teeth and gather the facts. Crate the emotional puppies and make a simple, logical assessment of the situation. Nuts and bolts. Pros and cons. Taking stock not only helps calm you down (What's the Flipside to anxiety? Focus!); it gives you a rough blueprint for dealing with it, when the time is right.

Principle #2: IDENTIFY YOUR REALISTIC IDEAL OUTCOME (RIO)

When shit happens, a full fix may or may not be possible, and that's okay. (I mean, it's gonna have to be.) You'll be far better off if you start with a realistic, achievable end goal in mind. The key to determining your RIO is to be honest with yourself. Honest about what's possible and what you want, honest about what you're capable of doing to get there, and honest about what's out of your control.

Think of it like buying a pair of shoes. When you try them on, no matter how much you like them, if they don't fit, they don't fit. Do not go to the cash register. Do not drop $200 on a pair of sweet-but-uncomfortable kicks.

You cannot will your size 10s to shrink overnight, and if the shoes pinch your feet now, imagine how your poor toes are going to feel after you walk around in them all day tomorrow.

Dealing with it becomes exponentially more difficult if you're chasing improbable outcomes and handicapping yourself with subpar tools.

Be realistic. Be honest with yourself. And be ready to walk away.

Comfortably.

Principle #3: TRIAGE

Triage is just a fancy word for prioritizing, which is at the heart of all of the advice I give. If a storm is already upon you, your probometer may have outlived its usefulness – but you can still prioritize based on urgency. Like an ER nurse, the faster you determine which patients are in the direst straits and which have the best chance of survival – i.e. which problems will get worse without your intercession and which stand the best chance of getting solved – the sooner you can minister effectively to each of them. You need to learn to do mental triage so you'll be prepared to deal when a total shitstorm blows through the swinging doors of your mental ER with little or no warning.

Dealing with it: a workshop

Think of the last bullshit thing that happened to you. Something that was out of your control. (Or maybe it was in your control but you didn't realize that in time and instead you just freaked out – whatever, you're learning.)

After it happened, how did you deal with it?

Knowing what you do now about the Three Principles of Dealing With It, what might you have done differently? And how might the outcome have changed?

....

....

....

....

....

....

....

....

....

....

....

....

....

....

Get bent! (A bonus principle)

When shit happens, it puts a minor-to-major dent in your plans. And while maintaining a rigid stance in the face of unwelcome developments such as these is good for, say, culling surprise Trump supporters from your Facebook feed, it's not terribly useful otherwise.

You gotta be FLEXIBLE.

I'm not talking about touching your nose to your hamstring (although that is impressive), but rather, you need to be able to regroup, reimagine, and reattack. Because when options seem to be closing off all around you, the ability to be flexible opens up new ones.

Remember: if you're still bending, you're not broken.

Make a list of shit that's happened lately where you being more flexible could have improved the outcome:

....

....

....

....

....

....

....

....

....

....

....

....

....

....

When you think of it that way, are you willing to try being more flexible in the future? Why or why not? (Hey, when it comes down to it, this is your life, your journal. You do you – and you live with the consequences.)

Whose fault is it anyway?

Placing blame is a classic impediment to dealing with whatever shit has happened. So much time wasted. So much energy. Why don't you take a unicycle ride across Appalachia while you're at it? Determining once and for all who was at fault doesn't fix your problem, and it won't make you feel better about it, either. How much satisfaction are you really going to get from browbeating your coworker Sven into admitting that he was the one who left the laptop with the presentation slides in the back of the taxi you shared last night? It's 7a.m., your client is expecting a PowerPoint bonanza in two hours, and you and Sven both smell like the back room at Juicy Lucy's. Put a pin in the blame game, hit the shower, and send Sven to the Staples in downtown Phoenix for some poster board and a pack of markers.

When was the last time you wasted time, energy, money, and/or goodwill by blaming someone else for shit that already happened, instead of just dealing with it?

....

....

....

....

....

....

Do you see the merit in putting a pin in it and spending your freakout funds on solutions instead? If not, why not?

....

....

....

....

....

....

Over to you, Bob

Congratulations! You are now in possession of a mental toolkit that you can apply (after the fact) to every possible iteration of all the shit that might and/or probably will happen to you.

In the original *Calm the Fuck Down*, I went through a lightning round of Relatively Painless Shit, Tedious Shit, and Really Heavy Shit that might and/or probably will happen to you, doling out my best advice along the way. It was pretty cool; maybe you should check it out someday.

But the *Calm the Fuck Down Journal* is for YOU. I'm just the foulmouthed, commonsense lady who's lighting the way.

Baby, it's your time to shine.

YOU
take stock of
what you see laid
out before you.

YOU
determine your
own realistic
ideal outcome.

YOU
set your
priorities and plans
in motion.

What the fuck just happened?

The final section of the journal is a place for you to flex your brand-new decision-making, problem-solving skills. The next time shit happens (and the next time, and the next time . . .), take to your journal!

- Work your Three Principles.

- Be flexible if the situation warrants.

- Waste not freakout funds on blame when you could be spending them on solutions.

- In other words: ORGANIZE your response.

THE NoWoRRIES METHOD

Step 1:

CALM THE FUCK DOWN

Step 2:

AND DEAL WITH IT.

What the fuck just happened?

....

....

Take stock

....

....

....

RIO

....

....

....

Triage

....

....

....

....

....

What the fuck just happened?

....

....

Take stock

....

....

....

....

RIO

....

....

....

Triage

....

....

....

....

....

What the fuck just happened?

....

....

Take stock

....

....

....

RIO

....

....

....

Triage

....

....

....

....

What the fuck just happened?

....
....

Take stock

....
....
....
....

RIO

....
....
....

Triage

....
....
....
....
....

What the fuck just happened?

Take stock

RIO

Triage

What the fuck just happened?

....

....

Take stock

....

....

....

RIO

....

....

Triage

....

....

....

....

What the fuck just happened?

....

....

Take stock

....

....

....

....

RIO

....

....

....

Triage

....

....

....

....

....

My Answers to the
Can I Control It? Quiz

What if I tell my bestie, Rachel, what I really think of her new bangs and she never forgives me?

Can I control it? Completely. Keep your trap shut and your friendship intact.

What if I accidentally shout another woman's name in bed with my new girlfriend?

Can I control it? Yes. For God's sake, Randy, get ahold of yourself. No wonder your new girlfriend doesn't trust you.

What if rumors of a union dispute come to pass and force the cancellation of that monster truck rally next Wednesday that I was all excited about?

Can I control it? Unless you also happen to be the Monster Truckers Union president, unequivocally no. Which means that this is a worry you should ideally DISCARD.

What if something bad happens to people I give incorrect directions to?

Can I control it? Yes, by telling the next nice young couple from Bismarck that you have a terrible sense of geography and they'd be better off querying a fire hydrant. This what-if is supremely easy to snuff out in its inception – take it from someone who thinks turning right automatically means going "east."

What if I laugh so hard I pee my pants during my friend's stand-up gig?

Can I control it? First of all, lucky you if your stand-up comedian friend is actually that funny. If you're prone to laugh-leaks, you may not be able to control the bladder, but you can make a contribution to your overall preparedness. There are many options in the personal hygiene aisle that were invented expressly to assist you in dealing with this issue.

I'm happy and in a good relationship, but what if we wait too long to get married and never have kids?

Can I control it? This is one you can heavily influence. You don't necessarily have full control over whether you get pregnant, but in terms of this specific what-if, you can control "not waiting too long" to start trying. You know how this whole aging-eggs thing works, and if you have to, you can explain it to Dan. However, if you have to explain it to Dan . . . maybe Dan should have paid more attention in tenth-grade bio.

What if I'm failing as an adult?

Can I control it? Yes. Adults do things like pay taxes, take responsibility for their actions, make their own dinner, and show up on time for prostate exams. Do these things and you will be succeeding as an adult. If your what-if is more existential in nature, perhaps you should get a hobby. Adults have those, too.

What if I choose not to go home and visit my family this weekend and something bad happens to them and then I regret it forever?

Can I control it? Yes. If your goal is not to have to worry about this, go visit them. If what you're really asking for is permission to not drive six hours to DC in holiday-weekend traffic and you also don't want to worry about the consequences of that decision, bust out your trusty probometer. How likely is it that something bad is going to happen to your family, this weekend of all weekends?

It's a Category 1, isn't it? You know what to do.

First published in Great Britain in 2019 by

Quercus Editions Ltd
Carmelite House
50 Victoria Embankment
London EC4Y 0DZ

An Hachette UK company

ISBN 978 1 52940 432 6

Some material previously published in *Calm the F**k Down*, also by Sarah Knight.

Illustrations and hand lettering by Lauren Harms

10 9 8 7 6 5 4 3 2 1

Designed and typeset by Carrdesignstudio.com

Printed and bound in Great Britain by Clays Ltd, Elcograf S.p.A.